Alzheimer And Dementia Disease

A Family Guide for Self-Care And Caring For Your Loved One

Patrick C. Lau

Copyright © 2024 by Patrick C. Lau

All rights reserved. No part of this book may be reproduced, distributed, or transmitted in any form or by any means, including photocopying, recording, or other electronic or mechanical methods, without the prior written permission of the publisher, except in the case of brief quotations embodied in critical reviews and certain other noncommercial uses permitted by copyright law. For permission requests, write to the publisher, addressed "Attention: Permissions Coordinator," at the address below.

TABLE OF CONTENT

Why You Need This Book 8
INTRODUCTION 12
CHAPTER 1 UNDERSTANDING DEMENTIA 16
   What Is Dementia? 16
   Types of Dementia 16
   Alzheimer's disease 18
   Vascular Dementia 20
   Lewy Body Dementia 21
   Frontotemporal Dementia 22
   Mixed Dementia 23
   Stages of Dementia 25
   Early Stage (Mild Dementia) 26
   Care Tips for the Early Stage 28
   Middle Stage (Moderate Dementia) 29
   Care Tips for the Middle Stage: 31
   Late Stage (Severe Dementia) 32
   Care Tips for the Late Stage 34
   Impact on Patients and Families 35
   Myths and Facts about Dementia 38
CHAPTER 2 DIAGNOSIS AND MEDICAL EVALUATION 44
   Seeking Medical Help 44
   Recognizing Early Signs and Symptoms 44
   Importance of Timely Intervention 46

Initiating the steps Towards Diagnosis 47

Involving Caregivers and Family Members 49

Comprehensive Evaluation Process 50

Conducting Initial Assessments Physical and Cognitive 50

Involvement of Caregivers and Family Members in Observations 52

Collaborating with Healthcare Professionals Neurologists, Psychiatrists, Geriatricians 53

Integrating Diagnostic Tests: MRIs, CT Scans, and Blood Tests 55

Understanding the Diagnosis: What's Next? 55

Emotional Responses and Coping Strategies 57

Educating Patients, Caregivers, and Families about Dementia 59

Planning for the Future Treatment Options, Care Plans, and Support Resources 60

Preparing for Lifestyle Adjustments 61

CHAPTER 3 MANAGING DAILY LIFE WITH DEMENTIA 64

Memory Aids and Tools 66

Technological Aids 67

Safety at Home: Fall Prevention and Emergency Preparedness 68

Nutrition and Meal Planning 70

Exercise and Physical Activity 73

Types of Exercise 74

Incorporating Exercise into Routine 75

CHAPTER 4 BEHAVIORAL AND PSYCHOLOGICAL SYMPTOMS 78

Understanding Behavioral Changes 78

Coping with Anxiety and Depression 80

    Strategies for Sleep Disturbances 82

    Dealing with Paranoia and Suspiciousness 84

CHAPTER 5 COMMUNICATION CHALLENGES 86

    Understanding Verbal and Non-verbal Cues 86

    Techniques for Effective Interaction 88

    Managing Communication Breakdowns 90

CHAPTER 6: LEGAL AND FINANCIAL PLANNING 96

    Importance of Early Planning 97

    Power of Attorney and Guardianship 98

    Understanding Insurance and Benefits 100

    Legal Considerations and Estate Planning 101

    Planning for Long-Term Care Costs 102

CHAPTER 7: SUPPORT SYSTEMS AND CAREGIVING 104

    Role of Caregivers 104

    Emotional and Physical Health of Caregivers 110

CHAPTER 8: LONG-TERM CARE OPTIONS 114

    In-Home Care vs. Residential Care 114

    Understanding Assisted Living and Nursing Homes 119

    Transitioning to Long-Term Care 121

    Specialized Dementia Care Units 125

CHAPTER 9: COPING STRATEGIES FOR FAMILIES 128

    Dealing with Grief and Loss 128

    Managing Family Dynamics 129

    Balancing Work and Caregiving Responsibilities 131

Preparing for the Future 133
CHAPTER 10: ADVANCES IN DEMENTIA RESEARCH 134
Current Trends in Dementia Research................................ 135
Promising Treatments and Therapies 136
Understanding Clinical Trials 137
Future Directions in Dementia Care 139
The Role of Genetics and Environmental Factors................ 140
Emerging Technologies in Dementia Care 141
Chapter 11: Prevention and Risk Reduction 142
Lifestyle Changes to Lower Risk... 142
The Importance of Diet and Exercise.................................. 143
Mental Stimulation and Cognitive Training 145
Cardiovascular Health and Dementia 146
Early Intervention Strategies 147
Social Engagement and Its Benefits................................... 148
CHAPTER 12: END-OF-LIFE CONSIDERATIONS 150
Recognizing the Final Stages of Dementia 150
Palliative and Hospice Care Options 152
Making End-of-Life Decisions... 154
Providing Comfort and Dignity 156
Supporting the Family During the Final Days..................... 158
Coping with Bereavement and Loss................................... 159
CHAPTER 13: LIVING WELL WITH DEMENTIA 162
Finding Moments of Joy and Connection 163

Celebrating Small Victories 165

The Power of Music and Art Therapy 166

CHAPTER 14: RESOURCES AND TOOLS 170

Apps and Technology for Dementia Care 170

Educational Programs and Workshops 173

Community and Government Resources 175

Tips for Staying Informed and Engaged 177

Creating a Personalized Care Plan 180

Why You Need This Book

Caring for a loved one with Alzheimer's or dementia is both a profound and challenging experience. "Alzheimer and Dementia Disease: A family Guide for Self-Care and Caring for Your Loved One" is an indispensable resource for several reasons:

Expert Guidance: Written by professionals with decades of experience, this book provides reliable, evidence-based advice tailored to the unique needs of dementia caregivers.

Comprehensive Coverage: From understanding the causes of dementia to managing early symptoms and providing care in the later stages, this book covers every aspect of the caregiving journey.

Practical Tips: Learn practical strategies to prevent caregiver burnout, manage daily activities, and cope with behavioral changes effectively.

Updated Information: Stay informed with the latest research and advancements in dementia care, including new therapies, technologies, and preventative techniques.

Supportive Insights: Gain emotional support and reassurance from compassionate advice, helping you navigate the emotional complexities of caregiving with confidence.

Easy Access: The user-friendly design allows you to quickly find the information you need, making it a handy reference for busy caregivers.

This book is more than just a guide; it's a lifeline, offering the tools and support you need to provide the best care possible while maintaining your own well-being.

Dear Reader,

Thank you for choosing "Alzheimer and Dementia Disease: A family Guide for Self-Care and Caring for Your Loved One." As you embark on this journey, know that you are not alone. This book is designed to provide you with the guidance, support, and practical advice you need to care for your loved one while also taking care of yourself.

Written by experts with decades of experience in the field, this book combines authoritative information with a compassionate approach to care. We understand the complexities and emotional challenges that come with caring for someone with memory loss, Alzheimer's, and other forms of dementia. Our goal is to equip you with the tools and knowledge necessary to navigate these challenges effectively.

This comprehensive guide covers everything from understanding the causes of dementia and managing its early stages to providing care in the later stages of the disease. We highlight useful takeaway messages and draw upon recent research to inform our recommendations.

In this book, you will find:

- **Brand-new content** on topics such as home care aides, useful apps, and promising preventative techniques and therapies.

- **Practical advice for avoiding caregiver burnout**, along with tips on when and how to seek additional help.

- A user-friendly two-column design that allows you to quickly access the information you need.

We have meticulously updated this edition to ensure it remains the most detailed and trusted resource available for caregivers. Our hope is that this book will not only provide you with practical strategies but also offer comfort and reassurance as you care for your loved one.

We deeply appreciate your commitment to providing the best care possible. Remember to take care of yourself, seek support when needed, and find moments of joy and connection along this journey.

INTRODUCTION

Caring for a loved one with Alzheimer's disease or any kind of dementia may be a challenging, stressful, and unpleasant experience. As a caregiver, you have the challenge of witnessing someone you care strongly about progressively change in ways that are difficult to comprehend and accept. The Alzheimer's and Dementia Disease book was written to navigate this challenging road, providing you with the knowledge, skills, and emotional support you need to unleash the greatest care while also looking after yourself.

Alzheimer's disease and other dementias are not limited to memory loss. They have an impact on all elements of a person's life, including the caregiver's. In quest of this book we made a thorough guide to understanding the neurological changes occurring in the brain as well as handling the day-to-day chores that can quickly become mammoth obstacles.

We will look at the complexities of dementia, helping you understand how the disease progresses and what changes to expect at each stage. You will learn about the many varieties of dementia, including Alzheimer's, and how they impact individuals. Knowledge is power, and understanding the disease will prepare you to face a variety of circumstances that may develop.

Daily chores that were once straightforward might become complicated and distressing for someone with dementia. As a caretaker, you must adjust to these changes and develop new methods to help your loved one navigate their day with dignity and independence as possible. This manual offers practical suggestions on how to manage everyday activities such as personal hygiene, dressing, eating, and movement. It is about providing a secure and supportive atmosphere in which both you and your loved one may thrive.

Behavioral changes are one of the most difficult aspects of dementia care. Your loved one may experience mood swings, anxiety, bewilderment, or even aggressiveness.

These behaviors can be upsetting and challenging to handle. We vividly simplify ways of dealing with these changes, focusing on patience, empathy, and clear communication. Learning how to respond to and control these behaviors will surely help you and your loved one feel less stressed.

The emotional impact of caring cannot be understated. Seeing someone you care about fade is distressing, and the obligations of caregiving may be daunting. It is critical to understand the value of self-care. Tools and suggestions on how to tackle and preserve your own health and well-being is what we reviewed making it easy and good for your own understanding, reminding you that in order to properly care for others, you must first take care of yourself.

Keep soaring in the book as each section will provide you with a combination of practical assistance, emotional support, and insightful information to assist you negotiates the challenges of dementia care. It is more than just a resource it's a companion on your caring process. You're not alone I have to assure that in the first place. Whether you are just starting out or have been on this process for a while, the Alzheimer's and Dementia is here for you as a caregiver it can be gifted to anyone who is the state of this disease. Together, we can make this memory an unforgettable and more bearable, meaningful, and full of opportunities for connection and love.

CHAPTER 1 UNDERSTANDING DEMENTIA

What Is Dementia?

Dementia is a broad term used to indicate a significant deterioration in cognitive function that interferes with everyday living and activities. It is a syndrome, not a single disease, which is a collection of symptoms caused by a variety of brain-related disorders or ailments. Memory, thinking, language, and other cognitive deficits are all characteristics of dementia. These alterations are usually progressive, which means they worsen with time.

Alzheimer's disease is the most prevalent kind of dementia, accounting for 60–80% of cases. Alzheimer's disease is characterized by the production of amyloid plaques and neurofibrillary tangles in the brain, which causes brain cell death.

Types of Dementia

While Alzheimer's disease is the most prevalent kind of dementia, other prominent varieties include vascular dementia, Lewy body dementia, and frontotemporal dementia. There are other uncommon forms of dementia caused by various illnesses and situations.

Mixed dementia occurs when a person develops different forms of dementia simultaneously. A younger individual may also get dementia. Young-onset dementia occurs when a person gets dementia before reaching the age of 65.

Dementia is not a single disease, but rather a broad term for a variety of cognitive deficits that interfere with daily activities. Understanding the various varieties of dementia allows caregivers and families to better manage and support their loved ones. We consider looking at the most prevalent types of dementia, such as Alzheimer's, Vascular, Lewy Body, and others.

Alzheimer's disease

Alzheimer's disease is the most prevalent kind of dementia, accounting for 60–80% of cases. It is distinguished by a progressive loss of memory and cognitive abilities. The illness proceeds through multiple phases, each characterized by increasing disability.

Early Stage: Symptoms are mild and may include forgetfulness, losing track of time, and becoming lost in familiar places.

Middle Stage: Memory loss and confusion become increasingly noticeable. Individuals may have trouble recognizing family and friends, experience significant changes in behavior, and need help with daily activities.

Late Stage: In the final stage, individuals lose the ability to communicate effectively, require full-time care, and may experience significant physical decline.

The exact cause of Alzheimer's is not fully understood, but it involves the buildup of amyloid plaques and tau tangles in the brain, leading to the death of brain cells.

Vascular Dementia

Vascular dementia is the second most common type of dementia, often resulting from strokes or other conditions that impair blood flow to the brain, leading to brain damage.

Symptoms: The symptoms can vary widely depending on the area and extent of brain damage. Common signs include problems with planning, organizing, and decision-making, as well as slower thinking and difficulty following the steps.

Progression: Vascular dementia often progresses in a stepwise manner, with sudden changes in cognitive ability following strokes or mini-strokes. Unlike Alzheimer's, the decline may not be as smooth or predictable.

Preventing strokes and managing cardiovascular health are important in reducing the risk of vascular dementia.

Lewy Body Dementia

Lewy Body Dementia (LBD) is characterized by the presence of Lewy bodies abnormal protein deposits in the brain. This type of dementia shares symptoms with both Alzheimer's and Parkinson's disease.

Symptoms: Common symptoms include visual hallucinations, fluctuating alertness, and attention, rigid muscles, and slow movement (similar to Parkinson's symptoms). Memory loss can also occur but is often less prominent in the early stages compared to Alzheimer's.

Progression: LBD tends to progress gradually, but cognitive fluctuations and motor symptoms can make the disease unpredictable and challenging to manage.

Early diagnosis is essential for managing symptoms and improving quality of life, as some medications for other types of dementia can worsen symptoms in LBD.

Frontotemporal Dementia

Frontotemporal Dementia (FTD) involves damage to the frontal and temporal lobes of the brain, areas associated with personality, behavior, and language.

Symptoms: Symptoms vary widely but can include dramatic changes in personality and behavior, impulsivity, and difficulty with language skills, such as speaking, writing, and comprehension.

Progression: FTD often develops earlier than other types of dementia, typically between the ages of 45 and 65. The progression can be rapid, with significant behavioral and language deterioration.

Because FTD affects younger individuals, the impact on families and caregivers can be particularly challenging, necessitating specialized support and resources.

Mixed Dementia

Mixed dementia refers to the presence of two or more types of dementia simultaneously. The most frequent combination is Alzheimer's disease and vascular dementia.

Symptoms: The symptoms of mixed dementia reflect the combined impact of each type involved, often leading to a broader range of cognitive impairments.

Progression: The progression can be more complex and variable, depending on the combination of underlying conditions.

Understanding that multiple factors contribute to cognitive decline will definitely be of good aid in developing comprehensive care plans that address the diverse needs of individuals with mixed dementia.

In all we are to consider that each type of dementia presents unique challenges and requires tailored approaches to care and management. By understanding the specific characteristics and progression of Alzheimer's, Vascular, Lewy Body, Frontotemporal, and Mixed Dementia, caregivers can better support their loved ones and navigate the complexities of these diseases.

Stages of Dementia

Dementia is a progressive condition, that's to say it worsens as time goes on. Understanding the stages of dementia can help caregivers and families anticipate changes and plan for the future. While the progression can vary depending on the type of dementia and the individual, it generally follows a pattern from mild to severe. Here, we explore the stages of dementia in depth, focusing on the characteristics and challenges of each phase.

Early Stage (Mild Dementia)

In the early stage of dementia, symptoms are often subtle and may be mistaken for normal aging. However, noticing these early signs is important for early diagnosis and intervention.

Memory Loss The most common early symptom is short-term memory loss. Individuals may forget recent events, appointments, or conversations, while long-term memories remain intact.

Confusion and Disorientation People may become easily confused about time or place, losing track of dates and misplacing items.

Difficulty with Complex Tasks: Managing finances, planning activities, or following a recipe can become challenging. Tasks that require multiple steps or strategic thinking may be particularly problematic.

Changes in Personality and Mood Individuals might experience mood swings, depression, or anxiety. They may become more withdrawn or show less interest in activities they previously enjoyed.

Communication Issues Finding the right words or following a conversation can be difficult, leading to frustration and social withdrawal.

Care Tips for the Early Stage

- Encourage participation in familiar activities to maintain skills and independence.

- Establish routines to provide structure and reduce confusion.

- Use memory aids like calendars, notes, and alarms to help manage daily tasks.

- Offer emotional support and promote social involvement.

Middle Stage (Moderate Dementia)

In the middle stage, the symptoms become more pronounced, and the individual requires more assistance with daily activities. This stage can be particularly challenging for caregivers as the need for support increases.

Increased Memory Loss: Memory issues become more severe, with individuals forgetting personal history, names of close family members, and recent events.

Behavioral and Psychological Symptoms: People may experience agitation, aggression, hallucinations, or delusions. They might wander, exhibit repetitive behaviors, or become suspicious of others.

Difficulty with Activities of Daily Living (ADLs): Assistance is often needed for tasks such as bathing, dressing, eating, and using the toilet.

Communication Breakdown: Language skills continue to decline, with individuals struggling to form coherent sentences or understand spoken and written language.

Loss of Orientation: Disorientation becomes more frequent, with individuals getting lost in familiar places or not recognizing their own home.

Care Tips for the Middle Stage:

- Create a safe environment by removing hazards and using locks or alarms to prevent wandering.

- Maintain a consistent daily routine to reduce confusion and anxiety.

- Use simple, clear communication and be patient when responding to repeated questions or behaviors.

- Seek support from healthcare professionals and consider joining support groups for caregivers.

Late Stage (Severe Dementia)

In the late stage of dementia, individuals become completely dependent on others for their care. The physical and cognitive decline is significant, and the focus shifts to providing comfort and maintaining quality of life.

Severe Cognitive Decline: Individuals lose the ability to communicate effectively, often speaking in short phrases or single words. They may not recognize loved ones or their surroundings.

Extreme Memory Loss: Almost all memory of past and recent events is lost. Individuals may not know their own identity.

Physical Decline: Mobility becomes severely impaired, with individuals often becoming bedridden. They may lose the ability to swallow, resulting in weight loss and increased risk of infections.

Incontinence: Loss of bladder and bowel control is common, requiring full-time care and management.

Behavioral Changes: While some individuals may become more passive, others might still experience agitation or distress.

Care Tips for the Late Stage

- Focus on comfort and dignity, ensuring the individual is as pain-free and relaxed as possible.

- Provide gentle physical care, including regular repositioning to prevent bedsores, and assist with feeding and hydration.

- Use sensory stimulation, such as music or gentle touch, to provide comfort and emotional connection.

- Seek hospice or palliative care services to support end-of-life needs and provide emotional support to the family.

Understanding these stages helps caregivers prepare and adapt to the evolving needs of their loved ones. By recognizing the symptoms and changes at each stage, caregivers can provide compassionate and effective care, ensuring the dignity and quality of life for individuals with dementia.

Impact on Patients and Families

The impact is multifaceted, encompassing emotional, practical, financial, and social challenges that require resilience, support, and understanding from all involved.

Emotional Impact

For patients, receiving a dementia diagnosis can evoke a range of emotions, from fear and confusion to grief and frustration. The gradual loss of cognitive abilities and independence can lead to feelings of helplessness, sadness, and a sense of identity loss. Patients may struggle to come to terms with their changing capabilities and the uncertainty of their future.

Families experience a similar emotional rollercoaster. They often juggle feelings of sadness, guilt, and anxiety as they witness their loved one's decline. The role reversal from being cared for to becoming a caregiver can be particularly challenging, triggering a mix of emotions and adjustments in family dynamics.

Practical Challenges

The practical challenges of dementia can be overwhelming. Patients may struggle with daily tasks such as dressing, eating, and personal hygiene, requiring increasing assistance as the disease progresses. This places a significant burden on caregivers, who must adapt to new caregiving responsibilities, manage medications, arrange appointments, and ensure a safe environment for their loved one.

Financial Strain

Dementia care comes with substantial financial costs, from medical expenses and medications to in-home care or assisted living facilities. Families often face difficult decisions about finances, long-term care planning, and navigating insurance or government assistance programs. The financial strain adds another layer of stress and complexity to an already challenging situation.

Social Isolation

Dementia can also lead to social isolation for both patients and caregivers. Stigma, misunderstanding, and the gradual withdrawal of the patient from social activities can contribute to feelings of loneliness and isolation. Caregivers may find their social circle shrinking as they prioritize caregiving responsibilities, leading to feelings of isolation and a lack of support.

Coping Strategies and Support

Despite the challenges, families impacted by dementia can find strength and flexibility through coping strategies and support networks. Open communication, education about the disease, and access to resources and support groups can help families pilot the emotional and practical aspects of caregiving. Seeking respite care, prioritizing self-care, and fostering meaningful connections with others facing similar challenges can provide much-needed support and validation.

Myths and Facts about Dementia

Unfortunately, numerous myths and misconceptions surround dementia, leading to stigma, fear, and misinformation.

We present to you some of the most prevalent myths about dementia and uncover the facts behind them.

Myth: Dementia is a process and Part of Aging

Fact: While aging is a risk factor for dementia, it is not an unavoidable aspect of growing old. Many elderly folks retain outstanding cognitive function far into their retirement years. Dementia is an illness, not a normal part of aging.

Myth: Memory Loss Equals Dementia

Fact: Memory loss can be a symptom of dementia, particularly in Alzheimer's disease. However, dementia encompasses a range of cognitive impairments beyond memory loss. These can include difficulties with language, problem-solving, decision-making, and changes in behavior and mood.

Myth: Dementia is Always Inherited

Fact: While genetics can play a role in some forms of dementia, such as early-onset Alzheimer's disease, most cases are not directly inherited. Environmental and lifestyle factors, such as cardiovascular health, education level, and social engagement, also influence dementia risk.

Myth: Nothing Can Be Done to Prevent Dementia

Fact: While there is no guaranteed way to prevent dementia, lifestyle factors can significantly impact risk. Engaging in regular physical activity, maintaining a healthy diet, staying mentally and socially active, managing chronic conditions like diabetes and hypertension, and avoiding smoking and excessive alcohol consumption can all contribute to brain health and potentially reduce dementia risk.

Myth: Dementia Only Affects Memory

Fact: Dementia affects multiple cognitive domains, including memory, language, executive function, attention, and visuospatial abilities. Individuals with dementia may experience a range of symptoms beyond memory loss, such as difficulty with communication, decision-making, and performing everyday tasks.

Myth: People with Dementia Are Violent and Aggressive

Fact: While behavioral changes can occur in some individuals with dementia, such as agitation or irritability, not everyone with dementia becomes violent or aggressive. These behaviors are often a result of the disease process and can be managed with appropriate care, understanding, and support.

Myth: Dementia is Untreatable

Fact: While there is currently no cure for most types of dementia, early diagnosis and intervention can significantly improve quality of life and slow disease progression. Medications, cognitive interventions, lifestyle modifications, and supportive therapies assist in managing symptoms and enhance well-being for individuals living with dementia and their caregivers.

Myth: People with Dementia Can't Learn Anything New

Fact: While dementia can impact learning and memory, individuals with dementia can still learn new skills and information, especially in the early stages of the disease. Adaptations such as repetition, visual aids, and simplified instructions can facilitate learning and engagement.

Myth: Dementia is Always Marked by Severe Memory Loss

Fact: While memory loss is a hallmark symptom of many dementias, including Alzheimer's disease, not all individuals with dementia experience severe memory impairment, especially in the early stages. Other cognitive changes, such as language difficulties, changes in behavior, or problems with executive function, may be more prominent initially.

Myth: Once Diagnosed with Dementia, is Life Over?

Fact: A dementia diagnosis is life-altering, but it does not signal the end of a worthwhile existence. Many individuals living with dementia continue to engage in activities they enjoy, maintain social connections, and find purpose and fulfillment. With appropriate support, education, and resources, life with dementia can still be rich and meaningful.

Keep moving slow steady as you are heading to the successful stage and be reminded that you are not alone

CHAPTER 2 DIAGNOSIS AND MEDICAL EVALUATION

Seeking Medical Help

Recognizing the early signs of dementia and seeking medical help is the first critical step in the stage towards diagnosis and management. Early intervention can significantly impact the quality of life and progression of the disease. See how you can handle this vital process.

Recognizing Early Signs and Symptoms

The symptoms often begin with noticing subtle changes in behavior, memory, and cognitive function. Common early signs of dementia include.

Memory Loss: Difficulty recalling recent events or significant facts.

Confusion: Frequently being lost or bewildered, especially in familiar surroundings.

Communication Issues: Struggling to find the right words, follow conversations, or complete sentences.

Mood and Personality Changes: Increased irritability, depression, anxiety, or a noticeable shift in personality.

Difficulty with Daily Tasks: Trouble with routine activities, such as managing finances, cooking, or driving.

Importance of Timely Intervention

Early medical intervention is always good for several reasons.

Accurate Diagnosis: Identifying dementia at an early stage allows for a more accurate diagnosis and differentiation between types of dementia.

Treatment and Management: Early diagnosis opens the door to treatments that can slow the progression of the disease and improve symptoms.

Planning for the Future Early awareness provides individuals and their family's time to plan for future care needs and make important decisions regarding legal, financial, and healthcare matters.

Support and Resources: Access to support groups, educational resources, and community services can be more readily obtained with an early diagnosis.

Initiating the steps Towards Diagnosis

1. **Consult Your Primary Care Physician**: The first step is to discuss any concerns with your primary care physician. They can conduct an initial evaluation and refer you to specialists if necessary.

2. **Prepare for the Appointment**: Before visiting the doctor, make a list of symptoms, changes in behavior, and any concerns. Include information about family medical history and any medications currently being taken.

3. **Undergo Initial Assessments**: The primary care physician will likely perform basic cognitive tests, review medical history, and conduct a physical examination. These initial assessments help determine if further evaluation is needed.

4. **Referral to Specialists**: Based on the initial findings, you may be referred to a neurologist, psychiatrist, or geriatrician for a comprehensive evaluation. Specialists have the expertise to

conduct more detailed tests and provide a definitive diagnosis.

Involving Caregivers and Family Members

Caregivers and family members play an important role in the medical evaluation process. They can provide additional insights and observations that are crucial for an accurate diagnosis. Their involvement includes:

Providing Detailed Observations Family members can describe changes in behavior, memory, and daily functioning that the individual may not notice or report.

Supporting During Appointments: Having a trusted person accompany the individual to medical appointments can provide emotional assistance and help in understanding and remembering the information provided by healthcare professionals.

Assisting with Communication Caregivers can help articulate concerns and questions, ensuring that all relevant information is communicated effectively to the healthcare provider.

Comprehensive Evaluation Process

A comprehensive evaluation process is nice for accurately diagnosing dementia and understanding its impact on an individual's cognitive and overall health. This process involves a series of detailed assessments conducted by healthcare professionals to gather a complete picture of the patient's condition.

Conducting Initial Assessments Physical and Cognitive

The comprehensive evaluation begins with initial assessments focusing on both physical and cognitive health.

Physical Examination: A thorough physical examination helps rule out other medical conditions that might mimic dementia symptoms. This includes checking vital signs, evaluating heart and lung function, and assessing general physical health.

Medical History: The healthcare provider will review the patient's medical history, including past illnesses, medications, and family history of dementia or other neurological conditions. This information helps identify potential risk factors and underlying causes.

Cognitive Testing: Cognitive tests are used to evaluate memory, problem-solving abilities, language skills, and other cognitive functions. Commonly used tests include the Mini-Mental State Examination (MMSE) and the Montreal Cognitive Assessment (MoCA). These tests provide a baseline measure of cognitive function and help track changes over time.

Involvement of Caregivers and Family Members in Observations

Caregivers and family members play a good role in the evaluation process. Their observations and insights provide valuable context and help healthcare professionals understand the patient's day-to-day challenges.

Behavioral Observations: Caregivers can report changes in behavior, mood, and daily functioning. These observations are essential for identifying patterns and triggers of dementia-related symptoms.

Functional Assessments: Information about the patient's ability to perform daily tasks, such as managing finances, cooking, and personal hygiene, helps assess the impact of cognitive decline on their independence.

Emotional and Social Changes: Family members can provide details about any changes in the patient's social interactions, emotional responses, and overall quality of life.

Collaborating with Healthcare Professionals Neurologists, Psychiatrists, Geriatricians

A multidisciplinary approach is often necessary for a comprehensive evaluation of dementia. Collaboration with specialists ensures a thorough and accurate diagnosis:

Neurologists: Neurologists specialize in disorders of the nervous system and are experts in diagnosing and managing dementia. They conduct detailed neurological exams, interpret brain imaging studies, and provide insights into the specific type and progression of dementia.

Psychiatrists assess the behavioral and psychological characteristics of dementia. They assess changes in mood, behavior, and mental health, providing support and treatment for conditions such as depression, anxiety, and agitation that often accompany dementia.

Geriatricians specialize in the health treatment of elderly persons. They address the complex medical needs of elderly patients, manage chronic conditions, and optimize overall health and well-being. Their expertise is invaluable in creating comprehensive care plans for individuals with dementia.

Integrating Diagnostic Tests: MRIs, CT Scans, and Blood Tests

Diagnostic tests are an integral part of the comprehensive evaluation process. These tests help confirm the diagnosis and provide detailed information about the brain's structure and function.

Imaging Studies MRI (Magnetic Resonance Imaging) and CT (Computed Tomography) scans provide detailed images of the brain. These imaging studies can detect structural abnormalities, brain atrophy, and other changes associated with different types of dementia.

Blood Tests: Blood tests are used to rule out other medical conditions that might cause or contribute to cognitive impairment. They can also identify biomarkers and genetic markers associated with specific types of dementia.

Understanding the Diagnosis: What's Next?

Receiving a dementia diagnosis can be a life-changing event, filled with a mix of emotions, questions, and uncertainties. Understanding what comes next is an important aspect of it for both the individual diagnosed and their loved ones. We stated the comprehensive guide to accessing the next steps after a dementia diagnosis

Emotional Responses and Coping Strategies

Emotional Reactions

Shock and Denial: It's common to feel shocked or in denial after receiving a dementia diagnosis. The reality of the condition can take time to process.

Fear and Anxiety: Concerns about the future, loss of independence, and changes in lifestyle may lead to fear and anxiety.

Sadness and Grief: Feelings of sadness and grief are natural as individuals and their families come to terms with the diagnosis.

Coping Strategies

Open Communication: Encourage open dialogue about the diagnosis. Sharing feelings and concerns with family members, friends, or support groups can be comforting.

Education: Learn about dementia, its progression, and what to expect. As knowledge in this aspect and every other aspect of life empower individuals and families to manage any kind of condition better.

Support Networks: Join support groups for individuals with dementia and their caregivers. These groups provide a sense of community and shared experiences.

Educating Patients, Caregivers, and Families about Dementia

Understanding the Disease

Progression: Dementia is a progressive condition, meaning symptoms will gradually get to tougher stage over time. Understanding the stages of dementia aids in anticipating changes and preparing for them

Symptoms Management: Learning about common symptoms such as memory loss, confusion, and behavioral changes enables better management and care.

Role of Caregivers

Active Involvement: Caregivers play a good role in providing support, managing daily activities, and ensuring the well-being of the individual with dementia.

Training and Resources: Caregivers should seek training and resources to improve their caregiving skills. Many organizations offer educational programs and materials.

Planning for the Future Treatment Options, Care Plans, and Support Resources

Treatment Options

Drugs: Although there is no cure for dementia, many drugs can help control symptoms and delay the development. Discussing these choices with healthcare practitioners is critical.

Therapies: Non-drug therapies, such as occupational therapy, cognitive stimulation, and physical exercise, can enhance quality of life and functional abilities.

Developing a Care Plan

Personalized Care: Create a care plan tailored to the individual's needs and preferences. This plan should include daily routines, medical appointments, and strategies for managing symptoms.

Legal and financial planning: it's always good to address legal and financial issues as early as possible.

This may include setting up power of attorney, creating advance directives, and planning for long-term care costs.

Accessing Support Resources

Community Services: Explore community resources such as adult day care centers, respite care services, and home care agencies. These services provide additional support and relief for caregivers.

Professional Help: Consider consulting social workers, case managers, or dementia care specialists who can offer guidance and connect families with appropriate resources.

Technology: Utilize technology and assistive devices to support daily living and enhance safety. Tools such as medication reminders, GPS trackers, and emergency response systems can be beneficial.

Preparing for Lifestyle Adjustments

Home Modifications

Safety: Make any required changes to the home to guarantee safety. This might involve adding grab bars, reducing tripping hazards, and enhancing illumination.

Comfort: Create a comfortable and familiar environment. Familiar objects and routines can help reduce anxiety and confusion.

Health and Wellness

Nutrition: Ensure a balanced diet to maintain overall health. Nutritional needs may change as dementia progresses, so adjustments to the diet may be necessary.

Physical Activity: Encourage regular physical activity to promote physical health and mental well-being. Tailor activities to the individual's abilities and preferences.

Social Engagement

Activities: Engage in meaningful activities that the individual enjoys. Maintaining social activity can enhance mood and cognitive performance.

Maintain solid ties with your family and friends. Social support is essential for emotional well-being and quality of life.

CHAPTER 3 MANAGING DAILY LIFE WITH DEMENTIA

Adapting to changes in daily routines is essential for individuals with dementia and their caregivers. As the disease progresses, maintaining a structured and predictable daily routine can help manage symptoms, reduce anxiety, and improve overall quality of life. Here are key aspects to consider.

Establishing a Routine

Consistency: Consistency is vital. Regular wake-up times, meal schedules, and bedtime routines provide a sense of stability.

Simplifying Tasks Break down tasks into simpler, manageable steps Use visual aids or written instructions to guide through each step

Flexibility: While consistency is important, flexibility is also a key. Be prepared to adjust routines based on the individual's needs and energy levels.

Involving the Individual

Engagement: Involve the individual in routine activities as much as possible. Participation focuses on a sense of autonomy and self-esteem.

Preferences: Consider personal preferences and past habits when creating routines. Familiar activities and environments can be comforting.

Memory Aids and Tools

Memory aids and tools can significantly assist individuals with dementia in managing daily activities and reducing frustration. We outline some effective strategies to follow.

Visual and Written Reminders

Calendars and Planners: Use large, easy-to-read calendars to mark important dates, appointments, and daily tasks.

Lists: Create checklists for daily activities, shopping, and household chores. Checklists provide a visual guide and sense of accomplishment.

Technological Aids

Digital Devices: Utilize smartphones, tablets, or digital assistants to set reminders and alarms for appointments and medications.

GPS Trackers: GPS tracking devices can help ensure safety by allowing caregivers to monitor the individual's location.

Voice Assistants: Devices like Amazon Echo or Google Home can offer reminders, answer questions, and provide entertainment.

Safety at Home: Fall Prevention and Emergency Preparedness

Ensuring safety at home is crucial for individuals with dementia. Fall prevention and emergency preparedness are key areas to address.

Fall Prevention

Clear Pathways: Remove clutter and ensure clear walking paths. Avoid using throw rugs or loose carpets that can cause tripping.

Grab Bars: Install grabs bars in bathrooms, hallways, and stairways to provide support and stability.

Ensure proper illumination in hallways, staircases, and bathrooms. Use nightlights to avoid falls on evening journeys.

Emergency Preparedness

Emergency Contacts: Keep a list of emergency contacts, including doctors, family members, and neighbors, in a visible location.

First Aid Kit: Maintain a well-stocked first aid kit and ensure everyone knows its location.

Emergency Plan: Develop an emergency plan that includes evacuation routes, meeting points, and procedures for different scenarios such as fires, natural disasters, or medical emergencies.

Nutrition and Meal Planning

Proper nutrition and meal planning are essential for maintaining health and well-being in individuals with dementia. Here come the strategies.

Balanced Diet

Variety: Provide a variety of foods to ensure a balanced diet that includes fruits, vegetables, whole grains, lean proteins, and healthy fats.

Hydration: Encourage frequent liquids intake to avoid dehydration.

Small, Frequent Meals: Serve small, frequent meals and snacks to maintain energy levels and prevent overeating or under reacting.

Simplifying Meals

Finger Foods: Offer easy-to-eat finger foods if using utensils becomes challenging.

Consistent Mealtimes: Maintain consistent mealtimes to establish routine and predictability.

Adaptive Utensils: Use adaptive utensils and dishes, such as plates with high edges or utensils with built-up handles, to assist with eating.

Personal Hygiene and Grooming

Maintaining personal hygiene and grooming can become challenging for individuals with dementia. Follow these tips to support activities.

Simplified Routines

Step-by-Step Instructions Provide step-by-step instructions for tasks such as brushing teeth, washing hands, and bathing.

Visual Aids Use pictures or diagrams to demonstrate each step of the hygiene routine.

Adaptive Equipment

Grab Bars and Shower Seats: Install grabs bar and use shower seats to ensure safety and comfort during bathing.

Electric Toothbrushes: Consider using electric toothbrushes, which can be easier to handle and more effective.

Exercise and Physical Activity

Regular exercise and physical activity are not to be overlook as it's important for maintaining physical health and mental well-being in individuals with dementia. We here by suggestion some types of exercises to take frequently.

Types of Exercise

Aerobic Exercise: Encourage activities such as walking, swimming, or dancing to promote cardiovascular health.

Strength training with resistance bands or modest weights helps preserve muscular mass and strength.

Flexibility and Balance Activities like yoga, tai chi, or simple stretching exercises can improve flexibility and balance.

Incorporating Exercise into Routine

Consistency: Aim for regular exercise sessions, ideally at the same time each day, to build routine and habit.

Engagement: Choose activities that the individual enjoys and finds engaging. This increases the likelihood of participation and enjoyment.

Coping with Sensory Changes

Individuals with dementia may experience changes in sensory perception, which can affect their interactions with the environment. Here are ways to manage these changes:

Vision and Hearing

Regular Check-ups: Schedule regular eye and hearing check-ups to address any issues and update prescriptions.

Adaptive Devices: Use adaptive devices such as glasses, magnifiers, or hearing aids to improve sensory function.

Creating a Sensory-Friendly Environment

Reduce Clutter: Minimize clutter to reduce visual distractions and create a calm environment.

Comfortable Lighting: Use soft, indirect lighting to create a comfortable ambiance. Avoid intense, bright lighting that may lead to discomfort.

Soothing Sounds: Incorporate soothing sounds or music to create a calming atmosphere. Avoid loud, sudden noises that can cause agitation.

Take a break; you can grab a cut of coffee while you assimilate what the book is all about, before continuation.

CHAPTER 4 BEHAVIORAL AND PSYCHOLOGICAL SYMPTOMS

Understanding Behavioral Changes

Behavioral changes in dementia are often a result of the brain's ongoing deterioration. These changes can vary widely and may include aggression, agitation, anxiety, depression, repetitive actions, sleep disturbances, hallucinations, delusions, paranoia, and suspiciousness. Recognizing that these behaviors are symptoms of the disease and not intentional acts can help caregivers respond with empathy and patience.

Managing Aggression and Agitation

Aggression and agitation are common in individuals with dementia and can be triggered by various factors, including physical discomfort, environmental stressors, or communication difficulties. Here are some ideas for managing these tendencies.

Identify Triggers: Pay attention to the circumstances that lead to aggressive or agitated behavior. Common triggers include noise, clutter, and changes in routine and physical discomfort.

Maintain a Calm Environment: Create a peaceful, structured environment. Reduce noise, minimize clutter, and establish a daily routine to help the person feel more secure.

Effective Communication: Use simple, clear language. Speak calmly and avoid arguing or correcting the person, as this can escalate the situation.

Physical Comfort: Ensure that the person is comfortable. Check for signs of pain, hunger, thirst, or the need to use the bathroom, as these can contribute to agitation.

Coping with Anxiety and Depression

Anxiety and sadness are common among dementia patients. These conditions can worsen cognitive symptoms and negatively impact quality of life. Ways to cope are here for you.

- **Routine and Structure:** Create a daily routine to increase predictability and security.

- **Engage in Activities:** Encourage participation in enjoyable and meaningful activities. Physical exercise, hobbies, and social interactions can improve mood and reduce anxiety.

- **Therapeutic Approaches:** Consider non-drug therapies such as music therapy, art therapy, or pet therapy, which can help alleviate anxiety and depression.

- **Professional Help:** Seek professional support from a psychologist or psychiatrist. Medications may be prescribed to manage severe anxiety or depression, but non-pharmacological approaches should be tried first.

Handling Repetitive Actions and Speech

Repetitive actions and speech, such as asking the same question repeatedly or pacing, are common in dementia. These behaviors can be challenging for caregivers but are usually harmless.

Respond with Patience: Answer repetitive questions calmly and consistently. Avoid expressing frustration or irritation.

Provide Distractions: Engage the person in a different activity to divert their attention. Simple tasks like folding laundry or looking through a photo album can be effective.

Create a Calm Environment: Reduce environmental stressors that may contribute to repetitive behaviors. A calm, structured environment can help.

Strategies for Sleep Disturbances

Sleep disturbances, including insomnia and nighttime wandering, are common in dementia and can significantly impact both the individual and their caregiver.

Establish a Routine: Maintain a regular sleep schedule with consistent bedtime and wake-up times.

Create a Relaxing Environment: Ensure the sleeping area is comfortable and conducive to sleep. Use nightlights to reduce disorientation if the person wakes up at night.

Limit Daytime Naps: Encourage daytime activities to reduce napping and promote nighttime sleep.

Monitor Your Diet and Exercise: Avoid coffee and big meals before bedtime. Regular physical exercise might help you sleep better. Addressing hallucinations and delusions.

Addressing Hallucinations and Delusions

Hallucinations (seeing or hearing things that are not there) and delusions (false beliefs) can be distressing for individuals with dementia and their caregivers.

Maintain Calm: Deal with hallucinations and delusions gently. Avoid arguing or trying to convince the person that their perceptions are incorrect.

Validate Feelings: Acknowledge the person's feelings without reinforcing the hallucination or delusion. For example, say, "That sounds frightening. I'm here with you."

Ensure Safety: Check that the surroundings is safe. Remove any objects that could cause harm if the person reacts to a hallucination or delusion.

Seek Medical Advice: Consult a healthcare provider if hallucinations or delusions become frequent or distressing. Medications may be necessary in some cases.

Dealing with Paranoia and Suspiciousness

Paranoia and suspiciousness can manifest as fear that others are stealing, spying, or planning harm. These feelings can stem from confusion and memory loss.

Reassurance: Offer reassurance and a calm presence. Validate their feelings without supporting false beliefs.

Consistent Environment: Maintain a consistent environment with familiar objects and routines to reduce confusion and anxiety.

Security Measures: Sometimes, practical measures such as keeping valuables in a secure place can help alleviate fears about theft.

Professional Support: Seek professional guidance if paranoia and suspiciousness significantly impact the person's well-being or caregiving becomes unmanageable.

Relax for 5-minutes after your coffee time to make a different that will shock you as you resume unto the next chapter of the book.

CHAPTER 5 COMMUNICATION CHALLENGES

Effective communication with a person who has dementia can significantly improve their quality of life and strengthen relationships. Understanding the nuances of verbal and non-verbal cues, employing effective interaction techniques, and managing communication breakdowns are essential skills for caregivers and loved ones. This chapter provides practical strategies to enhance communication, use technology to aid interaction, and engage in meaningful conversations with individuals living with dementia.

Understanding Verbal and Non-verbal Cues

Verbal Cues

Simple Language: Use clear, simple language and short sentences. Avoid complex words and long explanations.

Tone of Voice: Speak in a calm, reassuring tone. The tone of voice can convey warmth and understanding.

Repetition and Reinforcement: Repetition and reinforcement can help with comprehension. Be patient and give the other time to comprehend what you are saying.

Non-verbal Cues:

Body Language: Pay attention to body language, such as facial expressions, gestures, and posture. These cues can convey emotions and intentions.

Eye Contact: Maintain gentle eye contact to show attentiveness and engagement. However, be mindful that prolonged eye contact may be intimidating for some individuals.

Touch: A gentle touch on the hand or shoulder can provide comfort and reassurance, but always be aware of the person's comfort level with physical contact.

Techniques for Effective Interaction

Active Listening:

Full Attention: Give your full attention when the person is speaking. Make sure that you're paying attention by nodding, smiling, and saying things like I see or I understand.

Avoid Interrupting: Let the person express themselves without interruption. Interrupting can cause frustration and confusion.

Validation:

Acknowledge Feelings: Acknowledge and validate the person's feelings, even if their words don't make complete sense. When you alter words such as "I see you're upset" or "That sounds frustrating" might be soothing.

Redirecting If the person becomes agitated or confused, gently redirect the conversation to a more familiar or calming topic.

Use of Visual Aids:

Pictures and Objects: Use pictures, objects, or written cues to support communication. Visual aids can help clarify meaning and prompt memories.

Demonstrations: Demonstrate actions or tasks to help the person understand what you are communicating.

Managing Communication Breakdowns

Stay Calm and Patient

Remain Calm: Stay calm and patient when communication breaks down. Getting frustrated can increase the person's anxiety and confusion.

Rephrase and Repeat: If the person doesn't understand, rephrase the statement or question. Use simpler words and repeat as needed.

Minimize Distractions

Quiet Environment: Ensure the environment is quiet and free from distractions. Background noise can make it harder for the person to focus on the conversation.

One-on-One Interaction: Engage in one-on-one interactions rather than group conversations, which can be overwhelming.

Recognize Triggers:

Identify Triggers: Be aware of what might trigger communication breakdowns, such as fatigue, overstimulation, or emotional distress. Adjust your approach accordingly.

Provide Reassurance: Offer reassurance and a sense of safety if the person becomes upset or confused.

Using Technology to Aid Communication

Assistive Devices

Hearing Aids and Amplifiers: Ensure that hearing aids or sound amplifiers are working correctly. These technologies can help people hear and comprehend better.

Speech Generating Devices: Consider using speech-generating devices or apps that can assist in communication for individuals with advanced dementia.

Communication Apps

Visual and Text Aids: Use apps that provide visual and text aids to support communication. These can be particularly useful for people who have difficulty speaking.

Video Calls: Utilize video call technology to maintain connections with distant family and friends. Seeing familiar faces can be comforting and stimulating.

Reminiscence Therapy

Digital Photo Albums: Create digital photo albums or slideshows of meaningful memories and events. These can prompt conversations and evoke positive emotions.

Music Playlists: Curate playlists of favorite songs or music from the person's past. Music can be a powerful tool for triggering memories and enhancing mood.

Engaging in Meaningful Conversations

Personal Interests

Familiar Topics: Focus on topics that are familiar and interesting to the person. Discussing hobbies, favorite activities, or past experiences can engage them meaningfully.

Memory Sharing: Encourage the person to share their memories and stories. This not only improves cognitive performance but also offers a sense of belonging and approval.

Storytelling: Share stories from your own life or read aloud from books or articles. Narrating lots of story may be both soothing and engaging.

Reminiscence Therapy: Use reminiscence therapy techniques to stimulate memories and conversation. This can involve looking through old photos, discussing significant life events, or reminiscing about favorite places.

Positive Reinforcement:

Encouragement: Use positive reinforcement and encouragement in your talks. Recognize their attempts to communicate and offer thanks for their engagement.

Celebrate Small Successes: Celebrate small successes in communication, such as recalling a word or completing a sentence. This builds confidence and fosters a positive atmosphere.

Take a little time to write down exactly what your mind is telling you right now……..it's just time for you to do just that before you move on.

CHAPTER 6: LEGAL AND FINANCIAL PLANNING

Planning for the future is essential for individuals diagnosed with dementia and their families. Early and comprehensive planning can help manage the legal, financial, and healthcare aspects of living with dementia. Here we have covered the importance of early planning, power of attorney and guardianship, managing finances and assets, understanding insurance and benefits, legal considerations and estate planning, and planning for long-term care costs.

Importance of Early Planning

Early planning is critical following a dementia diagnosis. It ensures that the individual's preferences and best interests are respected and that the family is prepared for the future.

Proactive Decision-Making: Early planning allows individuals with dementia to make important decisions about their care, finances, and legal matters while they still have the cognitive ability to do so.

Reducing Stress Having a clear plan in place can reduce stress and uncertainty for both the individual and their caregivers.

Ensuring Continuity of Care: Planning ahead ensures that the individual's healthcare and personal care needs are met consistently, even as the disease progresses.

Power of Attorney and Guardianship

Power of attorney and guardianship are legal tools that allow someone to make decisions on behalf of an individual with dementia when they are no longer able to do so.

A Power of Attorney (POA) is a legal instrument that authorizes a trusted person (the agent) to make decisions on behalf of the individual (the principal). There are different types of POAs:

Durable POA: Stays in effect even if the primary becomes incompetent.

Healthcare POA: Allows the agent to make medical decision..

Financial POA: Grants the agent authority to manage financial affairs.

Guardianship: If no POA is in place and the individual with dementia becomes incapacitated, a court may appoint a guardian to make decisions on their behalf.

Guardianship might be more restricted, requiring regular court monitoring.

Managing Finances and Assets

Managing finances and assets becomes increasingly important as dementia progresses. It's essential to organize financial matters early to ensure stability and prevent potential issues.

Organize Financial Records: Gather and organize all financial records, including bank statements, investment accounts, bills, and tax returns.

Automatic Payments: Set up automatic payments for recurring bills to avoid missed payments and late fees.

Budgeting: Create a budget to manage day-to-day expenses and plan for future care costs.

Joint Accounts: Consider joint bank accounts to allow a trusted person to help manage finances if necessary.

Understanding Insurance and Benefits

Understanding insurance and benefits is crucial for covering medical expenses and accessing necessary care and support services.

Health Insurance: Review health insurance policies, including Medicare or Medicaid, to understand what is covered and any out-of-pocket costs.

Long-Term Care Insurance: If available, long-term care insurance can help cover the cost of care in a nursing home, assisted living facility, or at home.

Disability Benefits: Explore eligibility for disability benefits through Social Security or other programs.

Veterans Benefits: Veterans and their families may qualify for additional benefits and services through the Department of Veterans Affairs.

Legal Considerations and Estate Planning

Legal issues and estate planning guarantee that an individual's desires are followed and their possessions are safeguarded.

Wills and Trusts: Create or update a will to outline how assets should be distributed after death. Consider creating a trust to administer and preserve assets.

Advance directives, such as a living will, outline an individual's wishes for medical treatment and day-day life care.

Beneficiary Designations: Check and amend beneficiary designations for life insurance policies, retirement funds, and other financial assets.

Legal Advice: Consult with an elder law attorney to navigate complex legal issues and ensure all documents are properly prepared and executed.

Planning for Long-Term Care Costs

Planning for long-term care costs is essential, as dementia care can be expensive and extend over many years.

Assess Care Needs: Determine the type of care needed, whether it be in-home care, adult day care, assisted living, or nursing home care.

Cost Estimates: Research and estimate the costs of different types of care in your area.

Savings and Investments: Allocate savings and investments to cover future care costs. Consider liquidating assets or tapping into retirement funds if necessary.

Government Programs: Explore government programs, such as Medicaid, that may help cover the cost of long-term care.

Caregiver Support: Factor in potential costs for caregiver support services, including respite care and professional caregiving.

CHAPTER 7: SUPPORT SYSTEMS AND CAREGIVING

Caregivers often find themselves balancing multiple responsibilities while trying to provide the best possible care. Here we are to discuss various aspects of caregiving, emphasizing the importance of support networks, professional help, and maintaining the caregiver's own health and well-being.

Role of Caregivers

Caregivers play an important role in the lives of those who have dementia. Their responsibilities extend beyond basic daily care and include emotional support, medical management, and ensuring safety. Understanding the multifaceted role of caregivers can help in recognizing the breadth of their duties and the need for support.

Daily Care and Assistance:

Personal care includes helping with activities of daily living (ADLs) including bathing, dressing, eating, and toileting.

Medication Management: Ensuring that drugs are taken appropriately and on schedule.

Household Tasks: Managing household chores, preparing meals, and maintaining a clean and safe living environment.

Emotional Support:

Companionship: Offering emotional support and company to help people feel less alone and lonely.

Communication: Facilitating communication and helping the individual with dementia express their needs and feelings.

Medical Management:

Appointments: Scheduling and accompanying the person to medical appointments.

Monitoring Health Observing changes in health and behavior and communicating these to healthcare professionals.

Building a Support Network

A robust support network is essential for caregivers to sustain their caregiving efforts. Building a network involves seeking help from family, friends, and community resources.

Family and Friends

Delegating Tasks: Involve family members and friends in caregiving tasks. A little contribution will surely make a significant influence.

Emotional Support: Share feelings and experiences with trusted friends and family members to lighten the emotional load.

Community Resources:

Local Organizations: Many communities have organizations that offer services such as meal delivery, transportation, and in-home care assistance.

Faith-Based Groups: Religious or spiritual communities can provide emotional support, social interaction, and sometimes practical assistance.

Respite Care and Professional Help

Respite care and professional help are vital components of a caregiver's support system, providing relief and specialized care.

Respite Care:

Short-Term Relief: Respite care offers temporary relief for caregivers, allowing them to rest and recharge. This can be provided in-home or at specialized facilities.

Types of Respite Care: Options include in-home respite (care provided at home), adult day care centers, and residential respite care (short stays in a care facility).

Professional Help:

Home Health Aides: Trained professionals who assist with personal care, medical tasks, and household chores.

Nurses and Therapists: Healthcare professionals who provide medical care, physical therapy, and other specialized services.

Support Groups and Resources

Joining support groups and utilizing available resources can significantly enhance a caregiver's ability to manage their responsibilities and reduce feelings of isolation.

Support Groups

Peer Support: Support groups provide a platform for caregivers to share experiences, gain insights, and receive emotional support from peers who understand their challenges.

Educational Opportunities: Many support groups offer educational sessions on dementia care, stress management, and coping strategies.

Online Resources:

Websites and Forums: Numerous online resources offer information, advice, and community forums where caregivers can connect and share experiences.

Webinars and seminars: Online seminars and webinars offer essential information about dementia care and caring. Caregivers' Emotional and Physical Health

Emotional and Physical Health of Caregivers

Maintaining the emotional and physical health of caregivers is crucial for their well-being and their ability to provide effective care.

Emotional Health

Self-Care: Prioritize self-care by engaging in activities that promote relaxation and joy, such as hobbies, exercise, and socializing.

Professional Support: Seek counseling or therapy to address emotional challenges and mental health issues.

Physical Health

Regular Check-Ups: Caregivers must not overlook their own health. Regular medical examinations and preventative care are needed.

Healthy Lifestyle: Maintain a balanced diet, exercise regularly, and get adequate sleep to sustain physical health and energy levels.

Coping with Caregiver Stress and Burnout

Caregiving can be stressful and overwhelming, leading to burnout if not managed properly. Implementing coping strategies is essential to prevent and address caregiver stress.

Recognizing Burnout

Symptoms: Common signs of burnout include exhaustion, irritability, depression, and a sense of helplessness.

Awareness: Being aware of these symptoms and acknowledging them is the first step towards seeking help.

Stress Management Techniques:

Mindfulness and Relaxation: Practice mindfulness, meditation, and relaxation techniques to reduce stress.

Time Management: Organize and prioritize tasks to manage time effectively and reduce feelings of being overwhelmed.

Seeking Help

Professional Help: Don't hesitate to seek professional help, such as counseling or therapy, to address stress and burnout.

Support Systems: Lean on your support network for assistance and take advantage of respite care options.

CHAPTER 8: LONG-TERM CARE OPTIONS

In-Home Care vs. Residential Care

When faced with the issue of how to effectively care for a loved one with dementia, families frequently consider two major possibilities. in-home care and residential care. Each has its advantages and challenges, and the choice will depend on the individual needs of the patient and the family's circumstances.

In-Home Care

Familiar Setting: In-home care allows the individual to remain in a familiar environment, which may be reassuring and lessen confusion and anxiety.

Personalized Attention: Care can be tailored to the individual's specific needs, with one-on-one support from caregivers.

Flexibility: Families can adjust the level of care as needed, from a few hours a week to 24/7 support.

Challenges

Caregiver Stress: Family members often take on caregiving roles, which can lead to burnout and stress.

Limited Medical Care: In-home care might not provide the same level of medical supervision and emergency response as a residential facility.

Cost: Depending on the required level of care, in-home services can become expensive.

Residential Care

Comprehensive Care: Residential facilities offer a range of medical and personal care services, providing comprehensive support for individuals with dementia.

Social Interaction: Residents have opportunities to engage in social activities and build relationships with peers, which can enhance their quality of life.

Relief for Families: Knowing that their loved one is in a safe, controlled setting with competent care gives them piece of mind.

Challenges:

Adjustment Period: Transitioning to a residential facility can be challenging for the individual, requiring time to adapt to the new environment.

Cost: In-home services might be costly depending on the amount of care needed.

Limited Personalization: Care in residential facilities might be less personalized compared to in-home care, as caregivers manage multiple residents.

Choosing the Right Facility

Selecting the right care facility for a loved one with dementia is a significant decision. It involves careful consideration of various factors to ensure the facility meets the individual's needs and provides a supportive environment.

Key Considerations:

Level of Care: Assess the level of care required, from assisted living to skilled nursing care. Ensure the facility can accommodate current and future needs.

Staff credentials: Assess the staff's credentials and experience, including training in dementia care.

Facility Environment: Visit potential facilities to observe the environment, cleanliness, safety measures, and overall atmosphere.

Activities and Programs: Look for facilities that offer a variety of activities and programs tailored to individuals with dementia, promoting mental and physical well-being.

Location: Consider the facility's location in relation to family members and support networks to facilitate regular visits and involvement.

Questions to Ask:

- What is the staff-to-resident ratio?

- What specialized training do staff members have in dementia care?

- How does the facility handle medical emergencies?

- What types of activities and therapies are available for residents?

- What is the policy for family visits and engagement in care?

Understanding Assisted Living and Nursing Homes

Assisted Living:

Supportive Environment: Assisted living facilities provide a supportive environment for individuals who need help with daily activities but do not require intensive medical care.

Personalized Care Plans: Residents receive personalized care plans based on their specific needs, which may include assistance with bathing, dressing, medication management, and meal preparation.

Community Atmosphere: These facilities often foster a community atmosphere, with social activities, communal dining, and opportunities for residents to engage with peers.

Nursing Homes

Skilled Nursing Care: Nursing homes offer a higher level of medical care, with licensed nurses available around the clock to manage complex medical needs.

Comprehensive Services: In addition to personal care, nursing homes provide rehabilitation services, physical therapy, and access to medical specialists.

Secure Environment: Many nursing homes have specialized units for dementia care, offering a secure environment to prevent wandering and ensure resident safety.

Transitioning to Long-Term Care

Moving to a long-term care facility is a significant transition for individuals with dementia and their families. Preparing for this change can help ease the process and ensure a smoother adjustment.

Preparation Tips

Involve the Individual: Involve the person with dementia in the decision-making process as much as possible, respecting their preferences and concerns.

Familiar Items: Bring familiar items from home, such as photos, favorite blankets, and personal belongings, to create a sense of continuity and comfort.

Visit the Facility: Arrange visits to the facility before the move to help the individual become acquainted with the new environment and meet the staff and residents.

Communication: Maintain open communication with the facility's staff, sharing important information about the individual's routines, preferences, and medical history.

During the Transition:

Supportive Presence: Family members should be present during the initial days and weeks to provide reassurance and support.

Establish Routines: Work with the facility's staff to establish daily routines that mimic the individual's previous routines as closely as possible.

Monitor Adjustment: Keep an eye on how the individual is adjusting and address any concerns with the facility's staff promptly.

Maintaining Quality of Life in Care Facilities

Ensuring a high quality of life for individuals with dementia in care facilities involves focusing on their physical, emotional, and social well-being.

Physical Well-Being

Healthy Diet: Ensure that the institution serves healthy meals that meet the nutritional needs of the residents.

Regular Exercise: Encourage participation in physical activities and exercise programs to maintain physical health and mobility.

Regular medical check-ups and addressing health conditions are essential for preserving general well-being.

Emotional Well-Being

Mental Stimulation: Engage residents in mentally stimulating activities such as puzzles, reading, and memory exercises.

Emotional Support: Provide opportunities for residents to express their feelings and emotions, offering counseling or support groups if needed.

Comfort and Security: Create a comfortable and secure environment that minimizes stress and anxiety.

Social Well-Being

Social Interaction: Promote social interaction through group activities, events, and communal dining.

Family Involvement: Encourage regular visits from family and friends to maintain strong social connections.

Meaningful Activities: Offer activities that are meaningful and enjoyable to the residents, respecting their interests and preferences.

Specialized Dementia Care Units

Specialized dementia care units within residential facilities offer tailored care for individuals with advanced dementia. These units are designed to address the unique needs of dementia patients, providing a safe and supportive environment.

Key Features:

Secure Environment: Specialized units have enhanced security measures to prevent wandering and ensure the safety of residents.

Dementia-Specific Programs: Programs and activities are designed specifically for individuals with dementia, focusing on cognitive stimulation, sensory experiences, and emotional support.

Trained Staff: Staff members in these units are specially trained in dementia care, understanding the behaviors and needs of individuals with dementia.

Family Support: Specialized units often provide resources and support for families, helping them navigate the challenges of dementia care.

Benefits

Enhanced Quality of Life: Residents benefit from personalized care and activities that improve their quality of life.

Improved Safety: Enhanced security measures and staff training ensure a safe environment for residents with dementia.

Comprehensive Support: Families receive comprehensive support and guidance, helping them to cope with the progression of dementia.

What was the question you asked yourself back then?

Can you just remind yourself how progressive you are right now?

CHAPTER 9: COPING STRATEGIES FOR FAMILIES

Dealing with Grief and Loss

Acknowledging Emotions: Caregivers often experience a range of emotions, including sadness, anger, guilt, and grief. It's important to acknowledge these feelings and seek support from family, friends, or counseling services.

Coping Strategies: Engage in self-care practices such as mindfulness, journaling, or hobbies that bring comfort and relaxation. Participate in support groups where you can share experiences and learn coping strategies from others in similar situations.

Managing Family Dynamics

Open Communication: Initiate open communication within the family to address caregiving responsibilities, concerns, and decisions. Establishing defined responsibilities and expectations helps to avoid misunderstandings and confrontations.

Collaborative Decision-Making: Involve family members in decision-making processes related to care, finances, and future planning. Respect each person's input and seek consensus on important matters.

Educating and Involving Children and Teens

Age-Appropriate Education: Educate children and teens about dementia in age-appropriate ways. Provide simple explanations, answer questions honestly, and emphasize empathy and understanding towards the person with dementia.

Involvement in Care: Encourage children and teens to participate in caregiving activities suitable for their age and abilities. This may include spending time with the person with dementia, assisting with simple tasks, or creating meaningful interactions.

Balancing Work and Caregiving Responsibilities

Flexible Work Arrangements: Explore flexible work options such as telecommuting, flexible hours, or caregiver leave if available. Communicate with employers about your caregiving responsibilities and discuss potential accommodations.

Utilize Support Services: Seek support from community resources such as adult day care programs, respite care services, or professional caregivers to help manage caregiving duties while balancing work commitments.

Finding Joy and Meaning in the Caregiving processes

Focus on Moments of Connection: Cherish moments of joy and connection with the person with dementia. Engage in activities that bring smiles, laughter, and shared memories.

Self-Reflection: Take time for self-reflection and gratitude. Acknowledge the meaningful impact of caregiving and find purpose in providing love, support, and comfort to your loved one.

Preparing for the Future

Legal and Financial Planning: Review and update legal documents such as advance directives, power of attorney, and wills. Consider long-term care planning, including options for residential care if needed.

Self-Care and Support: Prioritize self-care to maintain physical, emotional, and mental well-being. Seek support from healthcare professionals, support groups, or counseling services as needed.

CHAPTER 10: ADVANCES IN DEMENTIA RESEARCH

Dementia research is continuously evolving, with new discoveries and innovations providing hope for better understanding, treatment, and care. This chapter delves into current trends in dementia research, promising treatments and therapies, the importance of clinical trials, future directions, the role of genetics and environmental factors, and emerging technologies in dementia care.

Current Trends in Dementia Research

Dementia research is a dynamic field focused on uncovering the underlying causes of the disease, identifying biomarkers for early detection, and developing effective treatments. Key trends include:

Neuroimaging: Advances in neuroimaging techniques, such as PET scans and MRI, allow researchers to visualize brain changes associated with dementia, aiding in early diagnosis and monitoring disease progression.

Biomarkers: Identifying biomarkers in blood, cerebrospinal fluid, and other tissues helps in early detection and tracking of dementia. Researchers are working on developing reliable biomarker tests for clinical use.

Genetics: Genetic studies are uncovering the role of specific genes in the development of dementia, providing insights into hereditary risk factors and potential targets for treatment.

Promising Treatments and Therapies

While there is currently no cure for dementia, several promising treatments and therapies are in development to slow disease progression, manage symptoms, and improve quality of life:

Drug Therapies: Researchers are investigating new drug therapies targeting amyloid plaques, tau tangles, and other pathological features of dementia. Some drugs aim to modify disease processes, while others focus on symptom management.

Immunotherapy: Immunotherapy approaches, such as vaccines and monoclonal antibodies, aim to stimulate the immune system to target and clear abnormal proteins associated with dementia.

Non-Pharmacological Therapies: Non-drug therapies, including cognitive training, physical exercise, and dietary interventions, are being studied for their potential to enhance cognitive function and overall well-being.

Understanding Clinical Trials

Clinical trials are very important for determining the safety and efficacy of novel treatments and therapies. Participating in clinical trials offers hope for individuals with dementia and contributes to scientific advancements:

Phases of Clinical Trials: Clinical trials typically progress through phases, starting with small-scale Phase I studies check safety, then Phase II trials analyze efficacy, and finally large-scale Phase III trials establish effectiveness and monitor adverse effects.

Eligibility and Enrollment: Each trial has specific eligibility criteria. Participants may undergo screening to determine their suitability for the study. Enrolling in clinical trials grants you access to cutting-edge therapies and thorough medical care.

Informed Consent: Participants provide informed consent, ensuring they understand the study's purpose, procedures, potential risks, and benefits. Ethical considerations and patient safety are paramount in clinical trials.

Future Directions in Dementia Care

The future of dementia care holds promise for improved diagnostics, treatments, and support systems. Emerging trends and innovative approaches are shaping the landscape of dementia care:

Personalized Medicine: Tailoring treatments based on individual genetic profiles, biomarkers, and disease characteristics offers the potential for more effective and targeted therapies.

Integrated Care Models: Holistic and integrated care models that address medical, psychological, and social needs are gaining traction. Coordinated care teams, including healthcare providers, social workers, and caregivers, ensure comprehensive support.

Telehealth and Remote Monitoring: Telehealth services and remote monitoring technologies enable continuous care and support, particularly for individuals in remote or underserved areas.

The Role of Genetics and Environmental Factors

Understanding the interplay between genetics and environmental factors is crucial in unraveling the complexities of dementia:

Genetic Risk Factors: Certain genes, such as APOE-e4, are associated with an increased risk of developing dementia. Genetic testing can provide insights into an individual's predisposition to the disease.

Environmental Influences: Lifestyle factors, including diet, physical activity, and exposure to toxins, play a significant role in dementia risk. Modifiable factors, such as cardiovascular health and cognitive engagement, can impact disease onset and progression.

Gene-Environment Interactions: Research is exploring how genetic and environmental factors interact, providing a comprehensive understanding of dementia's multifactorial nature.

Emerging Technologies in Dementia Care

Innovative technologies are transforming dementia care, offering new ways to enhance diagnosis, treatment, and support:

Artificial Intelligence (AI): AI algorithms analyze large datasets to identify patterns and predict disease progression. AI-powered tools assist in early diagnosis, personalized treatment planning, and monitoring cognitive changes.

Wearable technologies, including smart watches and fitness trackers, track vital indicators, physical activity, and sleep habits. These gadgets deliver real-time data to healthcare doctors and caregivers.

Assistive Technologies: Smart home systems, GPS trackers, and voice-activated assistants enhance safety and independence for individuals with dementia. These technologies offer reminders, emergency assistance, and remote monitoring.

Chapter 11: Prevention and Risk Reduction

Lifestyle Changes to Lower Risk

When you live a healthy lifestyle significantly it lowers the risk of developing dementia. By adopting certain habits and making conscious choices, you can promote brain health and reduce the likelihood of cognitive decline. Key areas to focus on include diet, exercise, mental stimulation, cardiovascular health, early intervention strategies, and social engagement.

The Importance of Diet and Exercise

Diet

Balanced Nutrition: A well-balanced diet rich in fruits, vegetables, whole grains, lean proteins, and healthy fats is essential for brain health. The Mediterranean diet, which focuses on fish, olive oil, almonds, and legumes, has been demonstrated to lower the risk of dementia.

Antioxidants and Omega-3s: Foods high in antioxidants (such as berries, leafy greens, and nuts) help protect brain cells from damage. Omega-3 fatty acids, found in fish like salmon and mackerel, support cognitive function and reduce inflammation.

Limit Sugar and Saturated Fats: High sugar intake and saturated fats can contribute to obesity, diabetes, and cardiovascular problems, all of which are risk factors for dementia. Cutting these short in diet can assist to preserve brain health.

Exercise

Regular Physical Activity: Engaging in regular physical exercise improves blood flow to the brain and encourages the growth of new brain cells. Prepare to exercise at least 150 minutes of moderate-intensity aerobic activity each week, for example brisk walking, swimming, or cycling.

Strength Training: Strength Training: make it mandatory to workouts twice a week. These exercises help maintain muscle mass, balance, and overall physical health, which are important for an active lifestyle.

Flexibility and Balance: Activities like yoga and tai chi improve flexibility and balance, reducing the risk of falls and injuries that can negatively impact overall health and mobility.

Mental Stimulation and Cognitive Training

Keep Your Brain Active:

Lifelong Learning: Continuously challenge your brain by learning new skills, hobbies, or languages. Educational activities stimulate brain function and create new neural connections.

Puzzles and Games: Engage in activities that require problem-solving, such as crossword puzzles, Sudoku, or strategy games. These activities keep your mind sharp and enhance cognitive abilities.

Reading and Writing: Regular reading and writing can help maintain cognitive function. Whether it's books, articles, or journals, these activities keep your brain engaged and improve memory.

Cardiovascular Health and Dementia

Heart-Brain Connection

Healthy Heart, Healthy Brain: Cardiovascular health is closely linked to brain health. Conditions like hypertension, diabetes, and high cholesterol can increase the risk of dementia.

Blood Pressure Management: Maintain healthy blood pressure levels through a balanced diet, regular exercise, and medications if prescribed. High blood pressure can damage blood vessels, leading to reduced blood flow to the brain.

Controlling cholesterol and diabetes: involves monitoring and managing blood sugar levels. High cholesterol can lead to plaque buildup in arteries, while diabetes can cause vascular damage, both contributing to dementia risk.

Early Intervention Strategies

Proactive Measures:

Schedule frequent medical check-ups to evaluate your general health and identify any possible problems early. Early detection of risk factors allows for timely intervention.

Screening for Cognitive Decline: Periodic cognitive screenings can help identify early signs of dementia. Early intervention with lifestyle changes and medical treatments can slow disease progression.

Stress Management: Chronic stress can have a harmful influence on brain health. Practice stress-reducing techniques such as mindfulness, meditation, deep breathing exercises, and yoga to maintain mental well-being.

Social Engagement and Its Benefits

Stay Connected

Meaningful Relationships: Maintain strong social connections with family, friends, and community. Social interactions stimulate cognitive function and provide emotional support.

Group Activities: Participate in group activities, clubs, or classes. Engaging with others in a social setting promotes mental health and prevents isolation.

Volunteer Work: Volunteering provides a sense of purpose and keeps you active and engaged. Helping others can improve your mood and overall well-being.

CHAPTER 12: END-OF-LIFE CONSIDERATIONS

As dementia progresses to its final stages, the focus of care shifts towards providing comfort, ensuring dignity, and supporting both the individual and their family. This chapter provides guidance on recognizing the final stages, exploring palliative and hospice care options, making end-of-life decisions, and coping with bereavement and loss.

Recognizing the Final Stages of Dementia

The final stages of dementia are characterized by significant cognitive and physical decline. Recognizing these changes is essential for preparing appropriate care and support.

Key Indicators:

Severe Cognitive Decline: Individuals may lose the ability to communicate, recognize loved ones, or understand their surroundings.

Physical Deterioration: There is often a marked decline in physical abilities, including difficulty swallowing, increased frailty, and profound weight loss.

Increased Dependence: Individuals become entirely dependent on others for daily activities such as eating, dressing, and personal hygiene.

Medical Complications: Increased susceptibility to infections, pressure ulcers, and other medical complications are common.

Palliative and Hospice Care Options

As dementia reaches its final stages, the emphasis shifts to palliative and hospice care, focusing on comfort and quality of life rather than curative treatments.

Palliative Care:

Palliative care addresses symptoms: including pain, shortness of breath, and agitation. This may involve drugs, treatments, and other interventions.

Holistic Approach: Care addresses physical, emotional, and spiritual needs, ensuring the individual's comfort and dignity.

Supportive Services: Palliative care teams offer support to both the individual and their family, providing resources and guidance during this challenging time.

Hospice Care:

Eligibility: Hospice treatment is usually considered when the life expectancy is six months or fewer. It focuses on providing compassionate end-of-life care.

Comprehensive Care: Hospice teams include doctors, nurses, social workers, chaplains, and volunteers who work together to provide comprehensive care.

In-Home and Facility-Based Options: Hospice care can be provided at home, in hospice facilities, or in nursing homes, depending on the individual's needs and preferences.

Making End-of-Life Decisions

End-of-life decisions are deeply personal and can be challenging. It is important to consider the individual's wishes, values, and beliefs.

Advance Directives:

Living Wills: A living will outlines the individual's preferences for medical treatments and interventions in the event they cannot communicate their wishes.

Durable Power of Attorney for Healthcare: This legal document designates a person to make healthcare decisions on behalf of the individual if they are unable to do so.

Discussions and Planning:

Open Conversations: Have open and honest discussions with family members, caregivers, and healthcare providers about end-of-life preferences and goals.

Respecting requests Ensure that the individual's requests are honored, and that their care plan is consistent with their values and beliefs.

Providing Comfort and Dignity

Ensuring comfort and dignity in the final stages of dementia is paramount. This includes providing a quiet and supportive environment.

Comfort Measures

Pain Management: Regularly assess and manage pain through medications and non-pharmacological methods.

Positioning and Mobility: Frequent repositioning and gentle exercises can help prevent pressure ulcers and discomfort.

Nutritional support: Serve small, regular meals and snacks that are simple to swallow and digest. Hydration is also important.

Dignity and Respect

Personal Care: Maintain personal hygiene and grooming to promote dignity and self-esteem.

Calm Environment: Create a calm and soothing environment with familiar objects, soft lighting, and comforting sounds.

Emotional Support: Offer reassurance, hold their hand, and speak in a gentle, soothing voice to provide emotional comfort.

Supporting the Family During the Final Days

Family members play a vital role during the final stages of dementia. Providing them with support and guidance is essential.

Emotional Support:

Counseling and Support Groups: Encourage family members to seek counseling or join support groups to share their experiences and feelings.

Respite Care: Offer respite care options to give family caregivers a break and time to rest.

Practical Assistance:

Information and Resources: Provide families with information about what to expect during the final stages and resources for managing care.

Coordination of Care: Help coordinate care among healthcare providers, hospice teams, and family members to ensure a seamless and supportive approach.

Coping with Bereavement and Loss

Coping with the loss of a loved one is a profound and personal journey. Grief can be complex, and finding ways to navigate this process is crucial.

Understanding Grief

Normal Reactions: Recognize that sadness is a natural and appropriate emotion to loss. It may involve a range of emotions, including sadness, anger, guilt, and relief.

Stages of Grief: Familiarize yourself with the stages of grief—denial, anger, bargaining, depression, and acceptance. Understand that these stages are not sequential and may differ from person to person.

Support Systems

Counseling and Therapy: Professional counseling and therapy can provide a safe space to process feelings and develop coping strategies.

Support Groups: Joining a support group can offer a sense of community and shared experiences, helping individuals feel less isolated in their grief.

Honoring Memories:

Memorials and Rituals: Participate in memorial services, rituals, or create personal memorials to honor and remember the loved one.

Journaling and Reflection: Writing down memories, thoughts, and feelings can be a therapeutic way to process grief and preserve cherished memories.

CHAPTER 13: LIVING WELL WITH DEMENTIA

Living in the moment is an essential practice for individuals with dementia and their caregivers. Focusing on the present helps reduce anxiety about the future and allows for meaningful, joyful experiences. Here, we explore how to embrace the present through various strategies, therapies, and community support.

Finding Moments of Joy and Connection

Engage in Meaningful Activities:

Hobbies and Interests: Encourage the individual to participate in activities they enjoy, whether it's gardening, painting, or reading. Familiar hobbies can provide a sense of purpose and achievement.

Daily Rituals: Establishing simple daily rituals, such as a morning coffee or an evening walk, can offer comfort and structure.

Promote Social Interaction

Spend meaningful time with your family and friends. Social interaction helps combat feelings of loneliness and depression.

Community Involvement: Participate in community events or support groups tailored for individuals with dementia. These gatherings provide opportunities for socialization and shared experiences.

Mindfulness and Relaxation

Mindfulness Practices: Techniques like deep breathing, meditation, and gentle yoga can help individuals stay grounded in the present moment.

Nature Therapy: Spending time outdoors and connecting with nature can be soothing and invigorating.

Celebrating Small Victories

Acknowledge Achievements

Daily Wins: Celebrate the small victories, such as remembering a name, completing a task, or enjoying a meal. These moments are significant and boost morale.

Positive Reinforcement: Use positive reinforcement to encourage and recognize efforts and accomplishments.

Set Realistic Goals

Short-term Goals: Focus on achievable short-term goals rather than long-term objectives. This approach keeps individuals motivated and provides a sense of accomplishment.

Adjust Expectations: Adapt expectations to match the individual's current abilities. Celebrate progress, no matter how small.

The Power of Music and Art Therapy

Music Therapy

Memory Stimulation: Music has the unique power to elicit memories and feelings. Listening to favorite songs or playing musical instruments can evoke positive feelings and memories.

Emotional Expression: Music therapy sessions allow individuals to express their emotions, reducing stress and enhancing mood.

Art Therapy

Art allows people to express themselves creatively. Painting, sketching, and crafts may be therapeutic as well as pleasurable.

Non-verbal Communication: Art therapy enables non-verbal communication, which can be particularly beneficial for those who have difficulty expressing themselves with words.

Building a Dementia-Friendly Community

Community Awareness

Education Programs: Implement community education programs to raise awareness about dementia and reduce stigma. Educated communities are more supportive and inclusive.

Dementia-Friendly Businesses: Encourage local businesses to become dementia-friendly by training staff to recognize and assist individuals with dementia.

Supportive Infrastructure

Accessible Environments: Create physical environments that are safe and accessible for individuals with dementia. This includes clear signage, good lighting, and safe walking paths.

Community Services: Develop community services that cater to the needs of individuals with dementia, such as memory cafes, support groups, and respite care options.

Adaptive Technologies for Daily Living

Assistive Devices:

Memory Aids: Utilize memory aids such as digital clocks, medication reminders, and labeled cabinets to support daily routines.

Safety Devices: Install safety devices like GPS trackers, emergency response systems, and fall detectors to ensure safety and provide peace of mind.

Smart Home Technology

Automated Systems: Implement smart home systems that control lighting, temperature, and appliances through voice commands or smartphone apps. These systems simplify daily tasks and enhance safety.

Monitoring Systems: Use monitoring systems that track movement and provide alerts to caregivers if unusual activity is detected.

Communication Tools:

Video Calls: Facilitate video calls with family and friends to maintain social connections, especially for those who may be isolated.

Simplified Phones: Provide easy-to-use phones with large buttons and simplified interfaces to assist with communication.

CHAPTER 14: RESOURCES AND TOOLS

Apps and Technology for Dementia Care

Technology has become an invaluable tool in managing dementia care. Various apps and devices are designed to help both individuals with dementia and their caregivers. This is how technology can make a difference

Memory Aids

Reminders and Alerts: Apps like Medisafe can help manage medication schedules, providing reminders to take medications on time.

Calendars: Digital calendars with alert features, such as Google Calendar, assist in keeping track of appointments and daily tasks.

Safety

GPS Trackers: Devices like GPS SmartSole or the Jiobit tracker can be worn discreetly, allowing caregivers to monitor the whereabouts of individuals with dementia and ensure their safety.

Emergency Response: Systems such as Life Alert or GreatCall's Lively Mobile offer emergency buttons that can summon help quickly if needed.

Cognitive Stimulation:

Brain Games: Apps like Lumosity and CogniFit offer cognitive exercises designed to improve memory and mental agility.

Virtual Reality: Tools like MyndVR use virtual reality to provide engaging experiences that can help stimulate cognitive function.

Communication:

Video Calling: Apps like Skype or Zoom enable easy video communication with family and friends, helping to maintain social connections and reduce feelings of isolation.

By integrating these technological solutions, caregivers can enhance the quality of care and safety for individuals with dementia.

Educational Programs and Workshops

Educational programs and workshops are essential for both caregivers and individuals with dementia. They provide knowledge, skills, and strategies to better manage the condition. Here are some significant advantages and possibilities.

Caregiver Training:

Skills Development: Programs offered by organizations like the Alzheimer's Association teach practical caregiving skills, such as managing daily activities, understanding behaviors, and effective communication techniques.

Stress Management: Workshops focus on stress reduction and self-care strategies for caregivers to prevent burnout.

Patient Engagement:

Cognitive Workshops: Programs designed for individuals with dementia, such as those by Memory

Cafés, provide activities that stimulate cognitive function and encourage social interaction.

Art and Music Therapy: Creative arts and music therapy sessions can be therapeutic and enhance quality of life by engaging senses and emotions.

Community Education

Awareness Campaigns: Local health departments and community centers often host events to raise awareness about dementia, its impact, and available resources.

Support Groups: Regular meetings with other caregivers and individuals affected by dementia can provide emotional support and practical advice.

Participating in these programs and workshops can significantly enhance the caregiving experience and improve the well-being of individuals with dementia.

Community and Government Resources

A variety of community and government resources are available to support families affected by dementia. These resources can provide financial assistance, respite care, and other essential services.

Community Resources:

Adult Day Care Centers: These centers offer structured activities and social interaction for individuals with dementia, providing a break for caregivers.

Respite Care Services: Temporary relief services, such as those provided by local senior centers or nonprofit organizations, allow caregivers to take a break while ensuring their loved ones are cared for.

Government Programs

Medicaid and Medicare: These programs offer various benefits; including coverage for certain medical services, in-home care, and long-term care facilities.

Area Agencies on Aging (AAA) These agencies provide a range of services, including meal programs, transportation, and case management for older adults, including those with dementia.

Nonprofit Organizations

Alzheimer's Association: Provides extensive resources, including a 24/7 helpline, support groups, and educational materials.

Dementia Care Central: Offers information on caregiving, financial planning, and legal issues related to dementia care.

By leveraging these resources, families can receive the support they need to navigate the challenges of dementia care.

Tips for Staying Informed and Engaged

Staying educated and active is good for providing successful dementia care. Here are some practical tips to help caregivers and individuals with dementia stay up-to-date and involved:

Stay Educated

Read Books and Articles: Regularly reading reputable sources on dementia can keep you informed about new research, treatments, and caregiving strategies.

Follow Trusted Organizations: Subscribe to newsletters and updates from organizations like the Alzheimer's Association to receive the latest information and resources.

Engage in Continuous Learning

Attend Workshops and Webinars: Participate in educational events to learn new caregiving techniques and connect with experts in the field.

Join Support Groups: Regular attendance at support groups can give continuous information and emotional assistance.

Utilize Online Resources

Websites and Blogs: Follow websites and blogs dedicated to dementia care for tips, personal stories, and expert advice.

Social Media: Join online communities on platforms like Facebook or Reddit where caregivers share experiences and resources.

Incorporate Technology

Health Monitoring Apps: Use apps to track health metrics and stay informed about the individual's well-being.

Online Forums: Engage in discussions on forums to share insights and learn from others in similar situations.

By staying informed and engaged, caregivers can provide better care and adapt to the evolving needs of individuals with dementia.

Creating a Personalized Care Plan

A personalized care plan is essential for managing dementia effectively. It should be personalized to each individual's specific needs and tastes, as well as flexible enough to change as the disease advances.

Assessment of Needs

Identify Daily Needs: Determine the individual's daily needs, including personal care, meals, and medication management.

Evaluate Abilities: Assess the individual's cognitive and physical abilities to create a plan that supports their independence while ensuring safety.

Setting Goals

Short-term Goals: Establish immediate goals, such as establishing daily routine or organizing medical appointments.

Long-term Goals: Plan for future needs, including legal and financial planning, potential residential care, and end-of-life care preferences.

Involving Caregivers

Roles and Responsibilities: Clearly define the roles and responsibilities of each caregiver to ensure all needs are met.

Backup Plan: Develop a backup plan for situations where the primary caregiver is unavailable.

Utilizing Resources

Community Services: Incorporate available community services, such as adult day care or respite care, into the care plan.

Professional Support: Hire geriatric care managers or social workers to give additional assistance and direction.

Regular Review and Adaptation

Monitor Progress: Review the care plan on a regular basis to ensure that the individual is making progress and making any required modifications.

Flexibility: Be prepared to adapt the plan as the individual's condition changes, ensuring it continues to meet their needs.

Creating a personalized care plan ensures comprehensive and coordinated care for individuals with dementia, enhancing their quality of life and providing peace of mind for caregivers.

By leveraging technology, engaging in educational programs, utilizing community and government resources, staying informed, and developing a personalized care plan, caregivers can effectively manage dementia and provide the best possible care for their loved ones.

www.ingramcontent.com/pod-product-compliance
Lightning Source LLC
Chambersburg PA
CBHW071920210526
45479CB00002B/487